FAT

BURNING

MASTERY

Unlock Your Body's Metabolic Potential to Achieve Optimal Health and Longevity

RYAN KLEIN

This book is intended to provide helpful and informative material on the subject matter covered. It is sold with the understanding that the author and publisher are not engaged in rendering medical, health, or any other kind of professional advice. If medical or health advice or other expert assistance is required, the services of a competent professional should be sought.

Neither the author nor the publisher shall be liable nor responsible for any loss or damage allegedly arising from any information or suggestions within this book.

Congratulations on writing such an insightful and informative book, "Fat Burning Mastery: Unlock Your Body's Metabolic Potential to Achieve Optimal Health and Longevity"! Your book is a must-read for anyone looking to improve their health and well-being through a better understanding of their body's metabolism.

Your thorough research and comprehensive approach to the topic are evident throughout the book, and your ability to explain complex concepts in a clear and accessible manner is truly impressive. Your writing stylc is cngaging and easy to follow, making it a pleasure to read from start to finish.

The practical tips and actionable advice you provide in "Fat Burning Mastery" are invaluable for anyone looking to improve their metabolic health, and your emphasis on the importance of long-term lifestyle changes is both refreshing and empowering.

Overall, "Fat Burning Mastery" is a must-have for anyone looking to take control of their health and unlock their body's metabolic potential. Your book is a true masterpiece, and I have no doubt it will inspire countless readers to make positive changes in their lives.

I believe your book will make a significant impact on the health and well-being of your readers. Your knowledge and expertise in the field of fat-burning and metabolic health are evident throughout the book. You have presented the information in an engaging and accessible manner that will resonate with a wide range of readers. Well done!

Sarah Ings

TABLE OF CONTENT

Introduction

Jennifer and her husband, Mike, had always struggled with their weight. They tried various diets and exercise programs, but nothing seemed to work for them. They were frustrated and disappointed and had almost given up hope of ever reaching their ideal weight.

One day, Jennifer came across one of my articles that talked about unlocking the body's potential to burn fat. She was intrigued and started researching more about it. She learned that the body has a natural ability to burn fat, but it can be hindered by various factors such as stress, lack of sleep, and poor diet.

Jennifer and Mike decided to give it a try and started implementing the tips they had learned. They started prioritizing sleep, reducing stress, and eating a healthy diet with plenty of whole foods and protein. They also started doing high-intensity interval training (HIIT) workouts, which are known to be effective for fat burning.

To their surprise, they started seeing results within a few weeks. They had more energy, felt less bloated, and their clothes were starting to fit better. They continued with their healthy lifestyle changes and before they knew it, they had both reached their ideal weight.

Jennifer and Mike were thrilled with their results and were amazed at how unlocking their body's potential had made such a difference in their weight loss journey. They felt healthier, happier, and more confident than ever before. They knew that this was not just a quick fix but a sustainable lifestyle change that they could maintain for the rest of their lives.

Understanding the Metabolic System

The metabolic system is a complex network of biochemical reactions that occur within living organisms to sustain life. These reactions involve the conversion of food into energy, the production of hormones and enzymes, and the elimination of waste products. Understanding the metabolic system is crucial for maintaining good health and preventing a variety of diseases, such as diabetes, obesity, and metabolic disorders. With advances in modern medicine and technology, researchers are gaining new insights into how the metabolic system functions, and how it can be optimized for optimal health.

The metabolic system plays a critical role in regulating various physiological processes, including growth, development, and reproduction.

It is responsible for converting the nutrients we consume into energy, which is then used to power the cells and tissues in our bodies. This energy is necessary for performing essential bodily functions, such as breathing, circulation, and digestion.

The metabolic system is comprised of several key components, including enzymes, hormones, and organs such as the liver, pancreas, and adipose tissue. Each component plays a unique role in the metabolic process, and disruptions to any one of these components can have significant effects on overall health and well-being.

For example, when the metabolic system is not functioning properly, it can lead to the development of conditions such as obesity, type 2 diabetes, and metabolic syndrome. These conditions are characterized by an imbalance in the body's metabolism, resulting in elevated levels of blood sugar, insulin resistance, and other metabolic abnormalities.

As our understanding of the metabolic system continues to evolve, so do our strategies for treating and preventing metabolic disorders. From diet and exercise to pharmaceutical interventions, there are a variety of approaches that can be taken to optimize metabolic health and reduce the risk of developing chronic diseases.

Understanding the metabolic system is essential for maintaining good health and preventing a variety of diseases. By gaining a deeper understanding of how this complex system works, we can develop new strategies for optimizing metabolic health and improving overall well-being.

This book will provide an overview of the metabolic system, including its key components, processes, and functions, to help readers gain a better understanding of this vital system.

Benefits of a Healthy Metabolism

A healthy metabolism is essential for maintaining good health and overall well-being. Metabolism refers to the process of converting food into energy, which is then used to fuel bodily functions such as breathing, circulation, and digestion. A healthy metabolism ensures that the body can efficiently break down food and convert it into energy, which can provide numerous benefits.

Here are some of the benefits of a healthy metabolism.

1. **Increased Energy Levels**: A healthy metabolism ensures that the body can efficiently convert food into energy. This means that individuals with a healthy metabolism are likely to have higher energy levels and feel less fatigued throughout the day.

2. **Weight Management:** A healthy metabolism can help individuals maintain a healthy weight. When the body can efficiently break down food and convert it into energy, excess calories are less likely to be stored as fat. This can help prevent weight gain and obesity.

3. **Improved Digestion**: A healthy metabolism can also improve digestion. When the body can efficiently break down

food, it can help prevent digestive issues such as constipation, bloating, and indigestion.

4. **Better Blood Sugar Control**: A healthy metabolism can also help regulate blood sugar levels. When the body can efficiently convert food into energy, it can help prevent spikes in blood sugar levels. This can be particularly beneficial for individuals with diabetes.

5. **Improved Mood:** A healthy metabolism can also improve mood. When the body can efficiently convert food into energy, it can help provide the brain with the fuel it needs to function properly. This can help improve mood and reduce feelings of anxiety and depression.

6. **Better Sleep:** A healthy metabolism can also improve sleep. When the body can efficiently convert food into energy, it can help provide the body with the energy it needs to repair and regenerate while sleeping. This can help improve sleep quality and reduce the risk of sleep-related disorders.

In conclusion, a healthy metabolism is essential for maintaining good health and overall well-being. By ensuring that the body can efficiently convert food into energy, a healthy metabolism can provide numerous benefits, including increased energy levels, weight management, improved digestion, better blood sugar control, improved mood, and better sleep.

Part I:

Foundations of Metabolic Health

Chapter 1

Nutrition for Optimal Metabolism

Nutrition plays a crucial role in maintaining optimal metabolism.

Here are some tips to consider for optimal metabolism:

1. **Eat a balanced diet**: A balanced diet that includes all the macronutrients (carbohydrates, proteins, and fats) and micronutrients (vitamins and minerals) in appropriate proportions is crucial for maintaining optimal metabolism.

2. **Stay hydrated:** Drinking enough water is important for maintaining a healthy metabolism. Dehydration can slow down metabolism and make it harder for the body to burn calories.

3. **Consume fiber-rich foods:** Fiber helps to slow down digestion and keep you feeling full for longer periods. This can help to regulate blood sugar levels and improve metabolism.

4. **Limit processed and sugary foods:** Processed and sugary foods can cause blood sugar spikes and crashes, which can negatively impact metabolism. Try to limit your consumption of these foods as much as possible.

5. **Include protein in your diet:** Protein helps to build and repair tissues in the body, and it also has a high thermic effect, which means that the body burns more calories digesting protein compared to fats and carbohydrates.

6. **Don't skip meals**: Skipping meals can slow down metabolism and make it harder for the body to burn calories. Aim to eat at least three meals per day and include healthy snacks as needed.

7. **Exercise regularly**: Exercise can help to boost metabolism and increase calorie burn. Aim for at least 30 minutes of moderate-intensity exercise per day.

8. **Get enough sleep:** Lack of sleep can disrupt metabolism and make it harder for the body to burn calories. Aim for at least 7-8 hours of sleep per night.

By following these tips, you can help to maintain optimal metabolism and improve overall health. However, it's important to remember that individual nutritional needs may vary depending on age, sex, activity level, and other factors. Consult a registered dietitian or healthcare professional for personalized advice.

The Role of Macronutrients

Macronutrients are essential nutrients that are required in large quantities by the human body to maintain normal growth, development, and overall health. The three macronutrients are carbohydrates, proteins, and fats.

1. **Carbohydrates**: Carbohydrates are the primary source of energy for the body. They are broken down into glucose and then used by the cells for energy. Good sources of carbohydrates include whole grains, fruits, vegetables, and legumes.

2. **Proteins**: Proteins are the building blocks of the body. They are essential for the growth, repair, and maintenance of tissues such as muscles, organs, and skin. Good sources of protein include meat, fish, eggs, dairy products, legumes, and nuts.

3. **Fats:** Fats are essential for various bodily functions such as insulation, cushioning of

organs, and absorption of certain vitamins. They are also a source of energy for the body. Good sources of fats include nuts, seeds, avocados, and fatty fish.

Each macronutrient plays a unique role in the body, and they all work together to maintain overall health. It is important to consume all three macronutrients in appropriate proportions to meet your individual needs and maintain a balanced diet.

The Power of Micronutrients

Micronutrients are essential nutrients that the human body requires in small amounts to function properly. These include vitamins, minerals, and trace elements. Despite their small quantities, they play a vital role in maintaining optimal health and preventing diseases.

Vitamins, for example, are organic compounds that are necessary for various metabolic processes in the body. They help with energy production, the formation of red blood cells, the maintenance of healthy skin and eyes, and the proper functioning of the immune system. Some common vitamins include vitamin C, vitamin A, vitamin D, and B vitamins.

Minerals, on the other hand, are inorganic substances that the body needs to carry out essential functions. These include maintaining healthy bones, regulating fluid balance, and supporting nerve and muscle function. Some common minerals include calcium, iron, zinc, and magnesium.

Trace elements are nutrients that are only needed in very small amounts but are still essential for good health. These include iodine, selenium, and copper.

The power of micronutrients lies in their ability to prevent nutrient deficiencies and promote overall health. Deficiencies in micronutrients can lead to a wide range of health problems, including anemia, weakened immune systems, and developmental delays in children. By ensuring that we consume adequate amounts of vitamins, minerals, and trace elements through a balanced diet or supplements, we can maintain optimal health and reduce the risk of chronic diseases.

Conclusively, micronutrients are essential for maintaining optimal health and preventing diseases. They play a vital role in various metabolic processes in the body, and deficiencies can lead to serious health problems. By ensuring that we consume a balanced diet rich in micronutrients, we can reap the benefits of optimal health and well-being.

Choosing the Right Foods

Nutrition is an essential component of a healthy lifestyle. It plays a crucial role in maintaining optimal metabolism and overall well-being. Choosing the right foods can help individuals achieve optimal nutrition and support their metabolism.

Optimal nutrition requires a balance of macronutrients and micronutrients. Macronutrients include carbohydrates, protein, and fats, while micronutrients include vitamins and minerals. Each of these nutrients plays a vital role in maintaining optimal metabolism and overall health.

Carbohydrates are the primary source of energy for the body. Choosing complex carbohydrates such as whole grains, fruits, and vegetables can help provide sustained energy and support metabolism. Simple carbohydrates, such as refined sugars and white bread, can cause blood sugar spikes and crashes, leading to metabolic imbalances.

Protein is essential for building and repairing tissues and maintaining muscle mass. Lean protein sources such as chicken, fish, beans, and lentils can provide essential amino acids and support metabolism. Avoiding processed meats and high-fat protein sources can help maintain a healthy weight and prevent metabolic imbalances.

Fats are essential for hormone production and nutrient absorption. Choosing healthy fats such as nuts, seeds, avocados, and olive oil can provide essential fatty acids and support optimal metabolism. Avoiding trans fats and saturated fats found in fried foods and processed snacks can prevent metabolic imbalances and promote overall health.

Micronutrients such as vitamins and minerals play a crucial role in supporting optimal metabolism. Choosing a variety of colorful fruits and vegetables can provide essential vitamins and minerals such as vitamin C, vitamin A, and potassium. Choosing whole grains and dairy products can provide essential minerals such as calcium and magnesium.

In conclusion, choosing the right foods can support optimal metabolism and overall health. A balanced diet rich in complex carbohydrates, lean protein, healthy fats, and essential micronutrients can help individuals achieve optimal nutrition and support their metabolism. Avoiding processed and high-fat foods can prevent metabolic imbalances and promote overall health.

Chapter 2

Movement for Metabolic Health

Engaging in regular physical activity and movement is an important factor in maintaining metabolic health. Metabolism refers to the chemical processes that occur within the body to convert food into energy, and regular exercise can help improve these processes.

Here are some body movements that can be beneficial for metabolic health:

1. **Strength Training**: Resistance training, such as weightlifting or bodyweight exercises, can help increase muscle mass and improve insulin sensitivity, which can

lead to better glucose control and a healthier metabolism.

2. **Aerobic Exercise**: Activities that increase heart rate and breathing rate, such as running, cycling, or dancing, can help burn calories and improve cardiovascular health. Regular aerobic exercise has been shown to improve insulin sensitivity and glucose control.

3. **High-Intensity Interval Training (HIIT):** HIIT involves short bursts of high-intensity exercise followed by periods of rest or low-intensity exercise. This type of exercise has been shown to increase metabolism and improve insulin sensitivity.

4. **Yoga**: Practicing yoga can help reduce stress levels, which can have a positive impact on metabolic health. Additionally, some yoga poses can help improve digestion and stimulate metabolism.

5. **Non-Exercise Activity Thermogenesis (NEAT)**: This refers to the energy expended through daily activities that are not considered exercise, such as walking, taking the stairs, or doing household chores. Increasing NEAT can help improve metabolic health and burn calories throughout the day.

It is important to consult with a healthcare provider before beginning any new exercise program, especially if you have any pre-existing medical conditions. Additionally, incorporating a balanced diet and healthy lifestyle habits, such as getting adequate sleep and managing stress levels, can also support metabolic health.

Exercise vs. Physical Activity

Exercise and physical activity are two terms that are often used interchangeably, but they have different meanings.

Physical activity refers to any movement of the body that requires energy expenditure. This can include activities such as walking, gardening, housework, or playing with your children.

Exercise, on the other hand, is a specific type of physical activity that is planned, structured, and repetitive, to improve one or more aspects of physical fitness, such as endurance, strength, or flexibility. Examples of exercises include running, weightlifting, or yoga.

While all exercises are physical activities, not all physical activities can be considered exercise. The key difference between the two is that exercise is typically done with a specific goal in mind, while physical activity can be done for various reasons, such as recreation or daily tasks.

Both exercise and physical activity are important for maintaining good health and preventing chronic diseases. It's recommended to aim for at least 150 minutes of moderate-intensity physical activity or 75 minutes of vigorous-intensity exercise per week, along with muscle-strengthening activities on two or more days per week.

The Importance of Resistance Training

Resistance training, also known as strength training or weight training, involves using resistance (such as weights or resistance bands) to build muscle and improve strength. It is an essential part of a well-rounded fitness routine and has many benefits for overall health and fitness.

Here are some key reasons why resistance training is important:

1. **Builds and maintains muscle mass**: Resistance training is an effective way to build and maintain muscle mass. As we

age, we naturally lose muscle mass, which can lead to weakness and frailty. By regularly engaging in resistance training, we can slow down this process and maintain our muscle mass, which helps us stay strong and healthy.

2. **Increases metabolism**: Muscle tissue is more metabolically active than fat tissue, meaning it burns more calories at rest. By building more muscle through resistance training, we can increase our metabolism and burn more calories throughout the day.

3. **Improves bone density**: Resistance training is a weight-bearing exercise, which means it places stress on the bones. This stress stimulates the bones to become

stronger and denser, which can help prevent osteoporosis and other bone-related conditions.

4. **Reduces the risk of injury**: Strengthening the muscles and connective tissues through resistance training can help reduce the risk of injury during exercise and in everyday life. Strong muscles provide better support for the joints and improve overall stability and balance.

5. **Improves overall fitness:** Resistance training can improve overall fitness by increasing strength, endurance, and flexibility. By challenging the muscles with resistance, we can improve our

ability to perform daily activities and other forms of exercise.

Overall, resistance training is an important component of a healthy and active lifestyle. It can help build and maintain muscle mass, increase metabolism, improve bone density, reduce the risk of injury, and improve overall fitness.

Incorporating Cardiovascular Exercise

Cardiovascular exercise, also known as cardio or aerobic exercise, is an important component of a healthy lifestyle. It can help improve cardiovascular health, increase endurance, and burn calories. Here are some tips for incorporating cardiovascular exercise into your routine:

1. **Start small:** If you're new to exercise or haven't done cardio in a while, start with small increments of exercise and gradually increase as you feel more comfortable. Even just 10 minutes of brisk walking or cycling can be beneficial.

2. **Mix it up:** Don't do the same type of cardio every day. Mix it up with different activities such as running, cycling, swimming, dancing, or jumping rope. This will keep things interesting and challenge your body in different ways.

3. **Find a buddy:** Exercise is more fun when you have someone to do it with. Find a

friend, or family member, or join a group class to stay motivated and accountable.

4. Schedule it in Make cardiovascular exercise a regular part of your schedule. Plan and find a time that works best for you, whether it's first thing in the morning, during lunch, or after work.

5. **Gradually increase intensity:** As you become more comfortable with cardiovascular exercise, gradually increase the intensity by adding intervals or increasing the resistance on a machine. This will help you challenge your body and continue to make progress.

Remember, it's important to consult with your healthcare provider before starting any new exercise routine, especially if you have any underlying health conditions or concerns.

Chapter 3

Sleep, Stress, and Metabolism

There is a complex relationship between sleep, stress, and metabolism. Sleep plays a crucial role in regulating metabolism, and chronic stress can disrupt sleep patterns, leading to metabolic dysfunction.

Here are some key points to consider:

1. **Sleep and metabolism:** Sleep deprivation can alter metabolism and increase the risk of obesity, insulin resistance, and diabetes. Lack of sleep can disrupt the balance of hormones involved in regulating appetites, such as leptin and ghrelin. This can lead to

increased food intake and weight gain. Moreover, sleep is critical for the body to carry out repair and maintenance functions, including tissue growth and repair.

2. **Stress and metabolism:** Chronic stress can lead to dysregulation of the stress hormone cortisol, which can interfere with metabolism. Cortisol can increase blood sugar levels, leading to insulin resistance and an increased risk of type 2 diabetes. Chronic stress can also increase inflammation, which is associated with many metabolic disorders.

3. **Sleep, stress, and metabolism**: Chronic stress can disrupt sleep patterns, leading to metabolic dysfunction. Sleep disturbances

can lead to dysregulation of the hormones involved in regulating appetite and metabolism, leading to weight gain and metabolic disorders.

In conclusion, getting adequate and quality sleep is crucial for maintaining a healthy metabolism, while chronic stress can disrupt sleep patterns and lead to metabolic dysfunction. It is important to prioritize sleep hygiene and stress management to promote optimal metabolic health.

The Connection Between Sleep and Metabolism

There is a close connection between sleep and metabolism, with research suggesting that getting adequate sleep is important for maintaining a healthy metabolism.

Sleep plays a critical role in regulating several hormones that influence metabolism, including leptin, ghrelin, insulin, and cortisol. Leptin is a hormone that suppresses appetite and helps to regulate energy balance, while ghrelin stimulates appetite and increases food intake. Sleep deprivation can reduce leptin levels and increase ghrelin levels, leading to increased hunger and food intake.

Sleep also affects insulin sensitivity, with sleep deprivation impairing insulin action and increasing the risk of developing insulin resistance and type 2 diabetes. Chronic sleep deprivation can also increase cortisol levels, a stress hormone that can promote the storage of fat and lead to weight gain.

Moreover, sleep plays a crucial role in the regulation of the circadian rhythm, which is the body's internal clock that regulates metabolism, digestion, and other physiological processes. Disruption of the circadian rhythm, such as with shift work or jet lag, can lead to metabolic disturbances and an increased risk of obesity and other metabolic disorders.

In summary, sleep and metabolism are closely linked, with adequate sleep playing a critical role in maintaining a healthy metabolism and preventing metabolic disorders.

The Impact of Chronic Stress

Chronic stress can have a significant impact on the human body's metabolism. The body's response to stress involves the release of hormones such as cortisol, which can affect metabolic processes.

Here are some of the ways chronic stress can impact metabolism:

1. **Increased blood sugar levels:** Chronic stress can cause the body to release glucose into the bloodstream, leading to

elevated blood sugar levels. Over time, this can increase the risk of developing type 2 diabetes.

2. **Increased appetite:** Stress can stimulate the release of appetite-stimulating hormones such as ghrelin, leading to an increase in food intake and potentially causing weight gain.

3. **Fat storage:** Chronic stress can also promote the storage of fat in the body, particularly in the abdominal area. This can increase the risk of metabolic syndrome and cardiovascular disease.

4. **Impaired insulin sensitivity**: Cortisol released during stress can impair the body's ability to use insulin, leading to

insulin resistance and potentially leading to type 2 diabetes.

5. **Slowed metabolism:** Chronic stress can cause the body to conserve energy, leading to a slowdown in metabolism. This can make it harder to lose weight and maintain a healthy weight.

6. **Hormonal imbalances**: Chronic stress can disrupt the balance of hormones in the body, leading to issues with the thyroid gland and sex hormones. This can affect metabolism and lead to a range of health problems.

Overall, chronic stress can have a significant impact on metabolism, potentially leading to a range of health problems. It is important to manage stress through healthy habits such as exercise, meditation, and stress reduction techniques to prevent these negative effects.

Strategies for Better Sleep and Stress Management.

Strategies for better sleep:

1. **Stick to a sleep schedule**: Go to bed and wake up at the same time every day, even on weekends.

2. **Create a relaxing bedtime routine:** Wind down before bed with relaxing activities such as reading, taking a bath, or practicing yoga.

3. **Avoid caffeine, nicotine, and alcohol:** These can interfere with sleep and lead to poorer quality sleep.

4. **Exercise regularly:** Regular exercise can improve sleep quality, but avoid exercising too close to bedtime as it can energize you and make it harder to fall asleep.

5. **Make your bedroom a sleep sanctuary:** Keep your bedroom cool, dark, and quiet. Use comfortable bedding and a supportive mattress and pillow.

6. **Limit screen time before bed:** The blue light emitted by screens can suppress melatonin production and disrupt sleep.

7. **Manage stress:** Stress and anxiety can keep you awake at night, so try relaxation techniques such as deep breathing, meditation, or progressive muscle relaxation.

Strategies for stress management:

1. **Identify your stressors:** Identity what causes you stress and try to avoid or manage those triggers.

2. **Practice relaxation techniques:** Relaxation techniques such as deep breathing, meditation, yoga, or tai chi can help you manage stress.

3. **Exercise regularly:** Regular exercise can reduce stress and anxiety.

4. **Prioritize self-care:** Take care of yourself by eating a healthy diet, getting enough sleep, and engaging in activities that you enjoy.

5. **Connect with others:** Spend time with friends and family, join a social group or volunteer in your community.

6. **Seek support:** Talk to a friend, family member, or mental health professional if you need help managing your stress.

7. **Practice time management:** Poor time management can lead to stress, so try to

prioritize your tasks and manage your time effectively.

Part II:

Unlocking Your Metabolic Potential

Chapter 4

Understanding Metabolic Resistance

Metabolic resistance, also known as metabolic adaptation, is a phenomenon that occurs when the body's metabolism slows down in response to a calorie deficit or increased physical activity. This can make it more difficult to lose weight or maintain weight loss over time.

When you reduce your calorie intake or increase your physical activity, your body may respond by slowing down your metabolism to conserve energy. This is a natural survival mechanism that has evolved over thousands of years to help our ancestors survive during times of famine and food scarcity.

However, in modern times, when food is readily available and physical activity is often limited, this metabolic response can work against us. If our metabolism slows down too much, it can make it difficult to lose weight or maintain weight loss over time, even if we continue to eat a healthy diet and exercise regularly.

Several factors can contribute to metabolic resistance, including genetics, age, hormonal imbalances, and certain medical conditions. Additionally, chronic stress, lack of sleep, and a diet that is too low in calories or too high in processed foods can all contribute to metabolic resistance.

To combat metabolic resistance, it's important to focus on maintaining a healthy diet, getting regular exercise, managing stress, and getting enough sleep. Additionally, it may be helpful to work with a healthcare professional or registered dietitian to develop a personalized plan that takes into account your unique needs and challenges.

What is Metabolic Resistance?

Metabolic resistance refers to a condition in which the body becomes resistant to the effects of certain hormones or neurotransmitters involved in metabolism. This can lead to a variety of metabolic disorders, including insulin resistance, leptin resistance, and thyroid resistance.

Insulin resistance is a condition in which the body's cells become resistant to the effects of insulin, a hormone that regulates blood sugar levels. This can lead to high blood sugar levels and eventually to type 2 diabetes.

Leptin resistance occurs when the body becomes resistant to the effects of the hormone leptin, which regulates appetite and energy expenditure. This can lead to overeating and weight gain.

Thyroid resistance occurs when the body becomes resistant to the effects of thyroid hormones, which regulate metabolism. This can lead to a slowing of the metabolism and weight gain.

Metabolic resistance can be caused by a variety of factors, including genetics, diet, lifestyle, and environmental factors. Treatment for metabolic resistance typically involves a combination of lifestyle changes, such as diet and exercise, and medication.

Causes of Metabolic Resistance

Metabolic resistance refers to a condition where the body's metabolism becomes less efficient at burning calories and can lead to difficulty in losing weight or maintaining weight loss. The causes of metabolic resistance can be multifactorial and complex and may include:

1. **Aging:** As we age, our metabolism slows down, and we tend to lose muscle mass, which can lead to a decrease in the number of calories burned at rest.

2. **Hormonal imbalances:** Hormones play a crucial role in regulating metabolism. Any hormonal imbalances, such as thyroid hormone imbalances, insulin resistance, or cortisol imbalances, can lead to metabolic resistance.

3. **Chronic inflammation:** Inflammation can interfere with the body's metabolic processes and lead to insulin resistance, which can impair the body's ability to burn fat.

4. **Poor diet:** A diet high in processed foods, sugar, and unhealthy fats can contribute to metabolic resistance by causing inflammation and disrupting the body's hormonal balance.

5. **Sedentary lifestyle:** Lack of physical activity can lead to a decrease in muscle mass and a slowing down of metabolism.

6. **Genetics:** Some people may be genetically predisposed to metabolic resistance, making it more difficult for them to lose weight.

7. **Medications:** Certain medications can affect metabolism and contribute to metabolic resistance.

8. **Sleep disturbances:** Lack of sleep or poor quality sleep can affect hormones that regulate metabolism and lead to metabolic resistance.

9. **Stress:** Chronic stress can disrupt hormonal balance and cause inflammation, which can contribute to metabolic resistance.

It's important to note that metabolic resistance can be a complex issue, and multiple factors can contribute to it. Therefore, addressing the underlying causes of metabolic resistance may require a multifaceted approach, which may include dietary changes, exercise, stress management, sleep hygiene, and medical treatment.

How to Overcome Metabolic Resistance

Metabolic resistance, also known as weight loss plateau, occurs when the body adapts to a certain level of exercise and diet, making it difficult to lose weight.

Here are some strategies to overcome metabolic resistance:

1. **Increase exercise intensity:** If you have been doing the same workout routine for a while, your body may have adapted to it. Increasing the intensity of your workouts can help you burn more calories and overcome metabolic resistance.

2. **Change up your exercise routine:** If you do the same exercises every day, your body may adapt to them and burn fewer calories. Try adding new exercises to your routine to challenge your body and keep it guessing.

3. **Reduce calorie intake:** As you lose weight, your body requires fewer calories to maintain its weight. Adjust your calorie intake accordingly to ensure you are in a caloric deficit and continue to lose weight.

4. **Increase protein intake:** Eating more protein can help you feel full and reduce your overall calorie intake. It also helps to maintain muscle mass, which is important for weight loss.

5. **Incorporate strength training:** Building muscle through strength training can increase your metabolism and help you burn more calories even at rest.

6. **Get enough sleep:** Sleep is essential for weight loss and metabolic function. Aim for at least seven hours of sleep per night to support your weight loss efforts.

7. **Manage stress:** Chronic stress can interfere with weight loss and metabolic function. Incorporate stress-reducing practices such as meditation, deep breathing, or yoga to support your weight loss goals. These practices have been shown to reduce cortisol levels and promote a sense of calm and relaxation,

which can help to counteract the negative effects of chronic stress.

Chapter 5

Intermittent Fasting for Metabolic Health

Intermittent fasting is a dietary strategy that involves restricting food intake for specific periods, to improve overall health and metabolic function. Several studies have suggested that intermittent fasting can have significant benefits for metabolic health, including:

1. **Improved insulin sensitivity:** Intermittent fasting has been shown to improve insulin sensitivity, which can help to lower blood sugar levels and reduce the risk of developing type 2 diabetes.

2. **Decreased inflammation**: Chronic inflammation is associated with several metabolic disorders, including insulin resistance and obesity. Intermittent fasting has been shown to reduce inflammation markers in the body, which may contribute to its metabolic benefits.

3. **Reduced oxidative stress:** Oxidative stress is a natural process that can damage cells and contribute to several metabolic disorders. Intermittent fasting has been shown to reduce oxidative stress, which may help to prevent or reduce the risk of metabolic diseases.

4. **Improved fat metabolism:** Intermittent fasting has been shown to improve fat

metabolism, which can help to reduce body fat and improve metabolic health.

Overall, intermittent fasting is a promising dietary strategy for improving metabolic health. However, it is important to note that it may not be suitable for everyone, particularly those with certain medical conditions or who are taking certain medications. It is always recommended to consult a healthcare professional before starting any new dietary or exercise regimen.

The Science Behind Intermittent Fasting

Intermittent fasting (IF) is a dietary approach that involves alternating periods of fasting and non-fasting. There are different variations of IF, but the most common types involve fasting for a certain number of hours per day or certain days of the week. The science behind IF suggests that it can have several health benefits, including weight loss, improved insulin sensitivity, and reduced inflammation.

One of the main ways IF works is by reducing calorie intake. By restricting the time window in which one can eat, individuals tend to eat less overall, which can result in weight loss. Additionally, during fasting periods, the body starts to break down stored fat for energy, which also contributes to weight loss.

IF has also been shown to improve insulin sensitivity, which is the body's ability to use insulin to regulate blood sugar levels. This is important because insulin resistance is a risk factor for several chronic diseases, including type 2 diabetes. During fasting periods, the body's insulin levels decrease, which can help improve insulin sensitivity over time.

Furthermore, research has shown that IF can reduce inflammation in the body. Chronic inflammation is associated with several health problems, including heart disease, cancer, and autoimmune disorders. Studies have found that IF can reduce the levels of pro-inflammatory markers in the body, which may help reduce the risk of developing these diseases.

In conclusion, the science behind intermittent fasting suggests that it can have several health benefits, including weight loss, improved insulin sensitivity, and reduced inflammation. However, it's important to note that IF is not suitable for everyone, especially those with certain medical conditions or who are pregnant or breastfeeding. It's always best to consult with a healthcare provider before starting any new dietary approach.

Different Approaches to Intermittent Fasting

Intermittent fasting (IF) is an eating pattern that involves cycles of eating and fasting periods. There are several different approaches to intermittent fasting, each with its unique benefits and effects on metabolism.

Here are some examples:

1. **Time-Restricted Feeding (TRF):** This approach involves restricting eating to a certain window of time each day, typically 8-12 hours. This can help regulate circadian rhythms and improve insulin sensitivity, which can lead to better metabolism and weight management.

2. **Alternate-Day Fasting (ADF):** ADF involves fasting every other day, with a normal eating pattern on non-fasting days. This approach has been shown to improve insulin sensitivity, decrease inflammation, and improve lipid metabolism.

3. **5:2 Diet:** This approach involves eating normally for five days of the week and restricting calories to 500-600 for two non-consecutive days of the week. This

can lead to improved insulin sensitivity, decreased inflammation, and weight loss.

4. **Extended Fasting:** Extended fasting involves abstaining from food for more than 24 hours, typically 48-72 hours. This can have a significant impact on metabolism, including improved insulin sensitivity, increased autophagy, and improved mitochondrial function.

Tips for Successful Fasting

Fasting can have several benefits for your overall health and well-being, but it can also be challenging, especially if you're new to it.

Here are some tips for successful fasting related to diet:

1. **Plan your meals:** Before starting your fast, plan your meals carefully. Ensure that you are consuming enough protein, fiber, and healthy fats to help you feel full for longer periods. Foods such as nuts, seeds, and whole grains are great for this.

2. **Stay hydrated:** It's essential to stay hydrated while fasting. Drink plenty of water throughout the day to help you feel full and reduce hunger pangs. You can also try herbal tea, sparkling water, or other non-caloric drinks.

3. **Choose nutrient-dense foods:** When you break your fast, focus on eating nutrient-dense foods that will provide your body with essential vitamins and

minerals. This will help you feel satisfied and reduce cravings.

4. **Start slowly:** If you're new to fasting, start slowly by gradually increasing the amount of time you fast. You can start with a 12-hour fast and gradually increase it to 16 or 24 hours as you become more comfortable.

5. **Listen to your body:** Pay attention to how your body feels during your fast. If you're feeling weak or lightheaded, it may be time to break your fast. Don't push yourself too hard and always prioritize your health.

6. **Stay busy:** When you're fasting, it's easy to get bored and think about food

constantly. Stay busy by engaging in activities that distract you, such as reading, exercising, or spending time with friends.

7. **Don't overeat:** When breaking your fast, avoid overeating. It's easy to get carried away and consume too many calories, which can negate the benefits of fasting. Instead, focus on eating slowly and mindfully, and stop when you feel satisfied.

Remember that fasting can be a personal experience, and what works for one person may not work for another. Experiment with different fasting schedules and find what works best for you. If you have any medical conditions or concerns, consult with a healthcare professional before starting a fasting regimen.

Chapter 6

The Benefits of Ketosis

Ketosis is a metabolic state in which your body starts to burn fat for energy instead of carbohydrates. This occurs when you limit your carbohydrate intake and increase your intake of fats and proteins.

There are several benefits associated with ketosis:

1. **Weight loss:** When your body is in ketosis, it burns stored fat for energy, which can lead to significant weight loss. Additionally, ketosis can help to reduce

hunger and cravings, making it easier to stick to a calorie-controlled diet.

2. **Improved blood sugar control:** By limiting your intake of carbohydrates, you can help to regulate your blood sugar levels. This is particularly beneficial for people with type 2 diabetes or insulin resistance.

3. **Reduced inflammation:** Ketosis has been shown to reduce inflammation in the body, which is associated with a range of health problems, including heart disease, cancer, and Alzheimer's disease.

4. **Increased energy:** Many people report feeling more energetic and mentally focused when in ketosis. This is because

the body is efficiently using fat for fuel instead of relying on carbohydrates.

5. **Improved physical performance:** Ketosis has been shown to improve physical performance in endurance athletes. This is because the body can efficiently use fat for fuel during exercise, which helps to conserve glycogen stores.

6. **Neuroprotective effects:** Ketosis has been shown to have neuroprotective effects, which may help to reduce the risk of neurological disorders such as Alzheimer's disease and Parkinson's disease.

Overall, ketosis can have numerous benefits for your health, including weight loss, improved blood sugar control, reduced inflammation, increased energy, improved physical performance, and neuroprotective effects. However, it is important to note that achieving and maintaining ketosis requires a strict dietary regimen and may not be appropriate for everyone. It is important to consult with a healthcare professional before making any significant dietary changes.

What is Ketosis?

Ketosis is a metabolic state in which the body uses ketones as a primary source of energy instead of glucose. This occurs when the body's carbohydrate stores are depleted, and it begins to break down stored fat for energy.

Ketones are molecules produced by the liver during the breakdown of fats, and they can be used by the body's cells as an alternative fuel source. In a state of ketosis, the body produces ketones in higher amounts, and they become the primary source of fuel for the brain and other organs.

Ketosis can occur naturally during fasting, prolonged exercise, or a low-carbohydrate, high-fat diet such as the ketogenic diet. It is often sought after as a weight-loss strategy because it can lead to increased fat-burning and reduced appetite. However, it can also have potential risks, particularly for individuals with certain medical conditions, and should be undertaken with caution under medical supervision.

How to Achieve Ketosis

Here are some steps to achieve ketosis:

1. **Reduce carbohydrate intake:** Limit your carbohydrate intake to 20-50 grams per day. This is the most crucial step to achieving ketosis, as it forces your body to switch from using glucose as its primary energy source to using ketones.

2. **Increase fat intake:** To replace the carbohydrates in your diet, you should increase your intake of healthy fats such as avocado, olive oil, coconut oil, and nuts.

3. **Moderate protein intake:** Protein should be consumed in moderation as too much

protein can also interfere with ketosis. Aim for 0.6 to 1 gram of protein per pound of body weight per day.

4. **Stay hydrated:** Drink plenty of water to keep your body hydrated and support ketone production.

5. **Exercise regularly:** Exercise helps deplete glycogen stores in the body, which is necessary for achieving ketosis.

6. **Use exogenous ketones:** Exogenous ketones can help speed up the process of entering ketosis, but they should not be relied upon as a long-term solution.

7. **Monitor your ketone levels:** You can monitor your ketone levels through blood,

urine, or breath tests to ensure that you are in ketosis.

It's important to note that achieving ketosis can have potential health risks and it's important to consult with a healthcare professional before starting a ketogenic diet.

The Benefits of a Ketogenic Diet

The ketogenic diet is a low-carbohydrate, high-fat diet that has gained popularity in recent years due to its potential health benefits. Here are some of the benefits of a ketogenic diet:

1. **Weight Loss:** One of the primary benefits of a ketogenic diet is weight loss. This is because the body burns fat for energy

instead of carbohydrates, leading to a reduction in body fat.

2. **Improved Blood Sugar Control:** A ketogenic diet can help improve blood sugar control, which is especially beneficial for individuals with type 2 diabetes. By reducing carbohydrate intake, the body's need for insulin decreases, leading to improved blood sugar levels.

3. **Increased Energy Levels:** Many people report increased energy levels when following a ketogenic diet. This is because the body is using fat for energy instead of carbohydrates, which can lead to sustained energy throughout the day.

4. **Improved Mental Clarity:** Some individuals report improved mental clarity and focus when following a ketogenic diet. This may be because the brain can use ketones (produced during ketosis) for energy.

5. **Reduced Inflammation:** Ketogenic diets have been shown to reduce inflammation in the body, which may lead to a reduction in chronic disease risk.

6. **Improved Cholesterol Levels:** Contrary to what many people believe, a ketogenic diet can improve cholesterol levels by increasing HDL (good) cholesterol and decreasing LDL (bad) cholesterol.

7. **Reduced Risk of Epileptic Seizures:** The ketogenic diet was originally developed as a treatment for epilepsy, and research has shown that it can significantly reduce the frequency and severity of seizures in individuals with epilepsy.

Overall, the ketogenic diet can be a powerful tool for improving health and well-being, particularly for individuals with obesity, type 2 diabetes, and epilepsy. However, it is important to speak with a healthcare provider before starting any new diet or making significant changes to your diet.

Part III:

Mastering Your Fat-Burning Potential

Chapter 7

The Power of Metabolic Flexibility

Metabolic flexibility refers to the body's ability to efficiently switch between using different fuel sources for energy production, such as glucose and fatty acids. This ability plays a crucial role in overall health and is increasingly being recognized as a key factor in preventing and managing chronic diseases.

When we consume food, the body breaks down the nutrients into various molecules that can be used for energy production. Glucose, for example, is a common energy source that comes from carbohydrates, while fatty acids come from dietary fats. The body also can produce glucose from non-carbohydrate sources, such as protein, through a process called gluconeogenesis.

In healthy individuals, the body can seamlessly switch between using glucose and fatty acids as fuel sources depending on the availability of nutrients and energy demands. This metabolic flexibility is important because it allows the body to maintain stable blood sugar levels, use stored fat for energy during periods of fasting or low carbohydrate intake, and avoid the negative effects of excess glucose and insulin resistance.

Research has shown that impaired metabolic flexibility is associated with a variety of health problems, including obesity, type 2 diabetes, and cardiovascular disease. Conversely, improving metabolic flexibility through lifestyle interventions such as diet and exercise has been shown to improve insulin sensitivity, reduce inflammation, and improve overall metabolic health.

In conclusion, metabolic flexibility is a key factor in overall health and can be improved through lifestyle interventions such as diet and exercise. By maintaining a healthy balance between glucose and fatty acid metabolism, we can optimize our body's ability to produce energy efficiently and reduce the risk of chronic diseases.

Understanding Metabolic Flexibility

Metabolic flexibility refers to the ability of cells, tissues, and organisms to adapt their metabolic pathways in response to changes in nutrient availability, energy demand, and physiological conditions. It is an essential aspect of metabolic homeostasis and plays a critical role in maintaining overall health and fitness.

At the cellular level, metabolic flexibility allows cells to switch between different energy substrates, such as glucose, fatty acids, and amino acids, to meet their energy needs. For example, during fasting or exercise, cells can utilize stored fats as an energy source instead of glucose. This ability to switch between different substrates is regulated by complex signaling pathways that involve hormones, transcription factors, and enzymes.

At the tissue and organismal level, metabolic flexibility is crucial for maintaining metabolic homeostasis in response to changes in nutrient availability and energy demand. For example, during periods of nutrient scarcity, metabolic flexibility allows the body to use stored energy reserves, such as glycogen and fat, to maintain energy balance and prevent starvation. In contrast, during periods of energy excess, metabolic flexibility allows the body to store excess energy in adipose tissue for later use.

Metabolic inflexibility, on the other hand, is a condition in which cells, tissues, or organisms are unable to adapt their metabolic pathways to changes in nutrient availability and energy demand. This can lead to metabolic dysfunction, insulin resistance, obesity, and other metabolic disorders.

Several factors can influence metabolic flexibility, including genetics, age, sex, diet, physical activity, and environmental factors.

Lifestyle interventions such as exercise and dietary modifications have been shown to improve metabolic flexibility and prevent metabolic disorders.

The Benefits of Metabolic Flexibility

Metabolic is the body's ability to switch between using different fuel sources (such as carbohydrates, fats, and proteins) for energy production, depending on the availability and demand for energy. Maintaining metabolic flexibility is important for overall health and well-being, and it offers a range of benefits, including:

1. **Improved energy levels:** When the body is metabolically flexible, it can use different fuel sources to produce energy,

which can help prevent energy crashes and keep you feeling energized throughout the day.

2. **Enhanced physical performance:** Metabolic flexibility can also improve athletic performance by allowing the body to switch between different fuel sources during exercise, depending on the intensity and duration of the activity.

3. **Better blood sugar control:** Metabolic flexibility helps the body regulate blood sugar levels by allowing it to switch between using glucose and fatty acids for energy, depending on the body's needs.

4. **Reduced inflammation**: Metabolic flexibility may help reduce inflammation

in the body by improving insulin sensitivity, which can help reduce the risk of chronic diseases such as type 2 diabetes and cardiovascular disease.

5. **Improved weight management:** Metabolic flexibility can also help with weight management by allowing the body to efficiently use stored fat for energy when glucose is not readily available, which can help promote fat loss.

Overall, maintaining metabolic flexibility through a healthy diet and regular exercise is crucial for optimal health and well-being.

How to Develop Metabolic Flexibility

Metabolic flexibility refers to the ability of the body to efficiently switch between different fuel sources, such as carbohydrates and fats, depending on the body's energy demands. Developing metabolic flexibility is important for maintaining overall health and managing weight.

Here are some ways to improve metabolic flexibility:

1. **Exercise regularly:** Exercise helps improve insulin sensitivity, which can enhance the body's ability to use glucose as fuel. It also helps increase

mitochondrial density and improve the body's capacity to burn fat as fuel.

2. **Follow a balanced diet**: A balanced diet that includes adequate amounts of protein, healthy fats, and complex carbohydrates can help improve metabolic flexibility. Additionally, intermittent fasting or time-restricted feeding can help improve insulin sensitivity and promote metabolic flexibility.

3. **Reduce stress:** Chronic stress can negatively impact metabolic flexibility by increasing cortisol levels, which can lead to insulin resistance. Therefore, reducing stress through techniques like meditation, yoga, or deep breathing exercises can help improve metabolic flexibility.

4. **Get enough sleep**: Sleep deprivation can impair glucose tolerance and insulin sensitivity, leading to decreased metabolic flexibility. Therefore, it is important to get adequate sleep to maintain metabolic health.

5. **Consider supplements**: Some supplements, such as omega-3 fatty acids, resveratrol, and berberine, may help improve metabolic flexibility. However, it is important to speak with a healthcare professional before adding any supplements to your routine.

In summary, improving metabolic flexibility requires a holistic approach that includes regular exercise, a balanced diet, stress management, adequate sleep, and possibly supplements. Making these changes can improve your overall health and help you maintain a healthy weight.

Chapter 8

Strategies for Sustainable Fat Loss

Several strategies can be helpful for sustainable fat loss:

1. **Create a calorie deficit:** The most important actor in fat loss is creating a calorie deficit, which means consuming fewer calories than your body needs. This can be achieved by reducing your portion sizes, choosing lower-calorie foods, and increasing your physical activity.

2. **Focus on whole foods:** Eating a diet that is high in whole, nutrient-dense foods such as fruits, vegetables, lean proteins,

and whole grains can help you feel full and satisfied while still reducing your overall calorie intake.

3. **Stay hydrated:** Drinking plenty of water can help keep you feeling full and reduce your appetite. It can also help support your body's natural fat-burning processes.

4. **Incorporate strength training:** Building muscle through strength training can help boost your metabolism and burn more calories, even when you're at rest.

5. **Find enjoyable forms of physical activity:** Regular exercise is important for sustainable fat loss, but it's also important to find activities that you enjoy and will

stick with. This could be anything from walking to yoga to weightlifting.

6. **Practice mindful eating:** Pay attention to your hunger and fullness cues, and try to eat slowly and mindfully. This can help you avoid overeating and make healthier food choices.

7. **Get enough sleep:** Getting adequate sleep is important for overall health, but it can also help regulate hormones that affect appetite and metabolism.

Remember, sustainable fat loss is a gradual process and requires consistency and patience. Focus on making small, sustainable changes to your lifestyle rather than trying to make drastic changes all at once.

The Truth About Quick Fixes

Quick fixes are often seen as easy solutions to problems that require more time, effort, and resources to solve. However, the truth about quick fixes is that they are usually temporary and may even make the problem worse in the long run.

Quick fixes are often band-aid solutions that address the symptoms of a problem, rather than the root cause. For example, taking painkillers may alleviate the pain temporarily, but it does not address the underlying health condition causing the pain.

Additionally, quick fixes can create a false sense of security and lead to complacency. People may become reliant on the quick fix and neglect to address the real issue, which can lead to more significant problems down the line.

In many cases, quick fixes are also not sustainable. They may work for a short period, but eventually, the problem will resurface, and the quick fix will no longer be effective.

To truly solve a problem, it is essential to address the root cause and take a more holistic approach. This may require more time, effort, and resources upfront, but it will lead to a more sustainable and long-lasting solution.

In summary, quick fixes may seem like an easy solution, but they are usually temporary, can make the problem worse, and create a false sense of security. To truly solve a problem, it is crucial to address the root cause and take a more holistic approach.

How to Set Realistic Goals

Setting realistic goals is crucial when it comes to achieving success in any area, including fat loss. Here are some steps to help you set realistic goals for fat loss:

1. **Start by assessing your current situation:** Before setting any goals, it's important to know where you're starting from. This includes determining your current weight, body fat percentage, and overall health. Consult with a healthcare professional if needed.

2. **Define your goal:** Determine what your desired outcome is for fat loss. Be specific and set a goal that is achievable within a certain timeframe. For example, your goal might be to lose 1-2 pounds per week over the next 12 weeks.

3. **Set realistic milestones:** Break your overall goal down into smaller milestones that you can achieve along the way. For example, if your overall goal is to lose 12 pounds in 12 weeks, set a milestone of losing 2 pounds per week.

4. **Make a plan:** Determine the steps you need to take to achieve your goal. This may include changes to your diet, exercise routine, and lifestyle habits. Be sure to

create a plan that is manageable and sustainable over the long term.

5. **Monitor your progress**: Keep track of your progress toward your goal. This can help you stay motivated and make adjustments to your plan if needed.

6. **Celebrate your successes:** When you reach a milestone or achieve your overall goal, take time to celebrate your success. This can help motivate you to continue making progress toward your next goal.

Remember, setting realistic goals is key to achieving success in fat loss. Be patient, stay consistent, and make adjustments as needed along the way.

Sustainable Lifestyle Changes for Fat Loss

Adopting sustainable lifestyle changes is key to achieving and maintaining fat loss. Here are some sustainable lifestyle changes you can make to support your fat loss goals:

1. **Eat a Balanced Diet:** A balanced diet that includes whole, nutrient-dense foods such as fruits, vegetables, lean proteins, and healthy fats can help you achieve and maintain fat loss. Avoid processed and junk food as much as possible.

2. **Practice Portion Control:** Eating the right amount of food is essential for fat loss. Using smaller plates, measuring your

food, and taking your time to eat can help you control your portions.

3. **Stay Hydrated:** Drinking plenty of water throughout the day can help boost your metabolism, reduce hunger, and support fat loss. Aim for at least 8-10 glasses of water daily.

4. **Move More:** Exercise is important for fat loss and overall health. Incorporating physical activity into your daily routine can help you burn calories, boost your metabolism, and build muscle mass.

5. **Get Enough Sleep:** Lack of sleep can disrupt hormones that regulate hunger and appetite, leading to overeating and weight gain. Aim for 7-8 hours of sleep per night.

6. **Reduce Stress:** Chronic stress can contribute to weight gain by increasing cortisol levels, which promotes fat storage. Practice stress-reducing techniques such as meditation, yoga, or deep breathing exercises.

7. **Seek Support:** Surround yourself with people who support your fat loss goals. Join a weight loss support group, hire a personal trainer or nutritionist, or enlist a friend to join you on your weight loss journey.

Remember, sustainable fat loss takes time and consistency. Make these lifestyle changes a part of your daily routine, and you'll be on your way to achieving your fat loss goals. Also, remember that sustainable fat loss is a journey, not a quick fix. By making these lifestyle changes a part of your daily routine, you can achieve your fat loss goals and maintain a healthy weight in the long term.

Chapter 9

Troubleshooting Your Metabolism

Metabolism refers to the chemical processes that occur within a living organism to maintain life. It is the process by which your body converts food into energy, which is then used to power various bodily functions.

If you feel like your metabolism isn't functioning properly, here are some troubleshooting tips:

1. **Eat enough protein**: Protein is essential for building and repairing tissues, and it can also help boost your metabolism. Make sure you're getting enough protein

in your diet by consuming foods such as meat, fish, eggs, beans, and nuts.

2. **Stay hydrated:** Dehydration can slow down your metabolism, so it's important to drink enough water throughout the day. Aim for at least 8 glasses of water per day.

3. **Exercise regularly:** Regular exercise can help boost your metabolism by building muscle mass and burning calories. Aim for at least 30 minutes of moderate-intensity exercise most days of the week.

4. **Get enough sleep:** Lack of sleep can disrupt your metabolism and make it harder for your body to burn calories. Aim for at least 7-8 hours of sleep per night.

5. **Reduce stress:** Stress can cause your body to release hormones that can slow down your metabolism. Find ways to reduce stress, such as through meditation, yoga, or other relaxation techniques.

6. **Eat a balanced diet:** Eating a balanced diet that includes a variety of fruits, vegetables, whole grains, and lean protein can help keep your metabolism functioning properly.

7. **Consider medical conditions:** Certain medical conditions, such as hypothyroidism or diabetes, can affect your metabolism. If you suspect you have a medical condition that is affecting your

metabolism, consult with your healthcare provider.

Common Pitfalls in Metabolic Health

Metabolic health refers to the state of metabolic processes within the body that influence overall health, including blood sugar regulation, lipid metabolism, and inflammation. Maintaining good metabolic health is important for preventing chronic diseases such as type 2 diabetes, cardiovascular disease, and obesity. However, there are several common pitfalls that people often encounter when trying to improve their metabolic health. Some of these pitfalls include:

1. **Relying on highly processed and refined foods:** Highly processed and refined foods often contain added sugars, unhealthy fats, and other additives that can contribute to insulin resistance and inflammation, two key factors that affect metabolic health.

2. **Skipping meals or going too long without eating:** Fasting or going too long without eating can lead to a drop in blood sugar levels and an increase in stress hormones, both of which can negatively impact metabolic health.

3. **Lack of physical activity:** Physical activity is important for maintaining healthy insulin sensitivity, which is essential for good metabolic health. Lack of exercise can contribute to insulin

resistance and increase the risk of chronic diseases.

4. **Chronic stress**: Chronic stress can lead to an increase in stress hormones like cortisol, which can negatively affect blood sugar regulation and contribute to inflammation, both of which can impact metabolic health.

5. **Lack of sleep:** Sleep is important for metabolic health, as it plays a role in regulating appetite hormones, insulin sensitivity, and inflammation. Chronic lack of sleep can lead to an increase in stress hormones, insulin resistance, and other negative effects on metabolic health.

6. **Overconsumption of alcohol:** Alcohol consumption can negatively impact metabolic health by contributing to insulin resistance, inflammation, and increased calorie intake.

7. **Not getting enough fiber**: Fiber is important for maintaining healthy blood sugar levels and regulating digestion. Lack of fiber can contribute to insulin resistance and other negative effects on metabolic health.

8. **Genetics:** While lifestyle factors can have a significant impact on metabolic health, genetics also play a role. Some people may be more susceptible to certain metabolic conditions due to their genetic makeup.

In conclusion, maintaining good metabolic health requires a holistic approach that involves a healthy diet, regular physical activity, adequate sleep, stress management, and other healthy lifestyle habits. By avoiding the common pitfalls listed above, you can improve your metabolic health and reduce your risk of chronic disease.

How to Identify and Overcome Plateaus

A plateau is a period during which you seem to make little or no progress toward your goals, despite putting in an effort. It can be frustrating and demotivating, but there are ways to identify and overcome it:

1. **Identify the plateau:** The first step is to recognize that you are on a plateau. This may be indicated by a lack of progress or improvement in your work, or a feeling of being stuck in a routine.

2. **Analyze the plateau:** Once you have identified the plateau, take some time to analyze it. What might be causing it? Is it a lack of motivation or a lack of knowledge/skills? Are there external factors that are hindering your progress?

3. **Set new goals:** If you have been working towards a particular goal for a while and have hit a plateau, it may be time to set new goals. This can help you regain focus and motivation and give you a sense of direction.

4. **Change your approach:** Sometimes, doing the same thing over and over again can lead to a plateau. Consider changing your approach to your work or finding new ways to challenge yourself.

5. **Seek feedback:** Getting feedback from others can help you identify areas where you may be falling short or could improve. It can also provide you with encouragement and support.

6. **Take a break:** Sometimes, taking a break from your work can help you gain a fresh perspective and come back with renewed energy and motivation.

Remember that plateaus are a natural part of the learning process and are often an opportunity for growth and improvement. Don't be discouraged by them, but rather see them as a chance to reassess your goals and approach to your work.

When to Seek Professional Help

If you are experiencing significant changes in your metabolism or related symptoms, it may be a good idea to seek professional help. Some signs that you may need to see a healthcare provider regarding your metabolism include:

1. **Significant weight gain or loss without a clear reason**: If you are experiencing unexplained changes in your weight, it could be a sign of an underlying metabolic issue.

2. **Fatigue and lethargy**: If you are feeling tired and sluggish even after getting enough rest, it could be a sign of an issue with your metabolism.

3. **Digestive issues:** Issues such as bloating, constipation, diarrhea, and other digestive problems may be a sign of a metabolic disorder.

4. **Hormonal imbalances:** If you are experiencing changes in your menstrual cycle, difficulty conceiving, or other hormonal issues, it could be a sign of an issue with your metabolism.

5. **Unusual cravings**: If you are experiencing unusual cravings for sugar or

salt, it could be a sign of an issue with your metabolism.

If you are experiencing any of these symptoms, it is important to see a healthcare provider to determine if there is an underlying issue with your metabolism. They may be able to provide a diagnosis and recommend a treatment plan to help you manage your symptoms and improve your overall health.

Conclusion

Maintaining Your Metabolic Health

Maintaining metabolic health is crucial for overall well-being and long-term health. Poor metabolic health can lead to various chronic diseases such as diabetes, cardiovascular disease, and obesity. To maintain metabolic health, it is essential to adopt a healthy lifestyle that includes regular physical activity, a balanced and nutritious diet, sufficient sleep, stress management, and avoiding harmful habits such as smoking and excessive alcohol consumption.

By implementing these lifestyle habits, you can promote healthy metabolism, regulate blood sugar levels, maintain a healthy weight, and reduce the risk of chronic diseases. It is also essential to prioritize regular medical check-ups to monitor metabolic health indicators such as blood pressure, blood glucose, and cholesterol levels. By detecting any metabolic health problems early, you can take appropriate measures to address them before they become more severe.

Overall, maintaining metabolic health is a long-term commitment that requires consistent effort and a holistic approach to health. By prioritizing your metabolic health, you can enjoy a better quality of life and reduce the risk of chronic diseases, ensuring that you can lead a healthy and fulfilling life.

In conclusion, "Unlock Your Body's Metabolic Potential to Achieve Optimal Health and

Longevity" is a guide to understanding how to optimize your metabolism for a healthier and longer life. By examining the latest research on metabolism and exploring the various factors that influence it, this book provides a comprehensive framework for achieving optimal metabolic health.

The book highlights the importance of proper nutrition, regular exercise, stress management, and sleep as essential elements of a healthy lifestyle. It also emphasizes the role of genetics, environment, and lifestyle in shaping an individual's metabolic profile.

Through practical tips and actionable advice, this book equips readers with the tools they need to take control of their metabolic health and achieve their wellness goals. Whether you are looking to lose weight, improve your energy levels, or prevent chronic diseases, "Unlock Your Body's Metabolic Potential to Achieve Optimal Health and Longevity" is an essential resource for anyone looking to improve their overall health and well-being.